The Compl Psilocybin Mushroom Blueprint

The A-Z Companion Guide To Growing And Using Magic Mushrooms

Arlie Williams

Introduction

Do you want to better unlock your creative faculties?

Do you want to take a break from your chaotic routine and promote relaxation throughout your body and mind?

Do you want to tap into your spirituality and unlock the state of intuition?

If yes, and you wish to enjoy all of that through organic means, 'magic mushrooms' are the perfect antidote for your needs. Found all across the globe and being revered by many cultures, magic mushrooms are a sacred and special specie of mushrooms that is known to relax users and activate a state of mysticism that helps users transcend beyond time and space, and better comprehend things.

While magic mushrooms are illegal in many countries and states, they are allowed to be cultivated in some states of the U.S.

If you want to learn how to cultivate magic mushrooms from scratch at home, this guide is for you.

It will walk you through the entire cultivation process step by step, leaving nothing to chance, to ensure you have your very own fresh supply of magic mushrooms to use in whichever way you want.

That's not all; the book will give insight into the power and benefits of magic mushrooms; how growing it can help you; and offers valuable, actionable and potent tips and tricks to grow them on your own.

To benefit well from this guide, it is important to gather all the supplies and equipment as the book guides you and follow the guidelines in a step by step manner as illustrated here. This way, you progress gradually and can correct on any mistakes on time instead of identifying and correcting them later on when the process is over.

Let's begin the journey.

Table of Contents

Introduction _____ 2

Chapter 1: Magic Mushrooms 101 _____ 8

What Are Magic Mushrooms? _____ 8

History Of Magic Mushrooms _____ 10

What Are The Other Names Of Magic Mushrooms? _____ 12

What Are The Uses Of Psilocybin Mushrooms? 12

*What Do Psilocybin Mushrooms Look Like?*___ 13

*How Are Magic Mushrooms Used?*_____ 14

How Do The Magic Mushrooms Taste? _____ 14

What Do Magic Shrooms Do To Your Body To Bring Their Effects? _____ 14

*What Are The Common Side-Effects Of Magic Mushrooms?*_____ 16

Chapter 2: Effects And Side Effects Of Magic Mushrooms _____ 18

What Happens When You Consume Psilocybin Mushrooms?_____18

What Is A Psychedelic Experience? _____ 21

How Magic Shrooms Interact With Different Food Items And Drugs _____ 22

Effects Of Magic Mushrooms By Dose _____ 23

Benefits Of Psychedelic Mushrooms _____ 33

Chapter 3: Growing Magic Mushrooms With Ready To Use Kits _____ 42

Psilocybin Mushroom Ready To Grow Kit With Substrate _____ 42

Growing Magic Shrooms Using Mushroom Spawn Bags _____ 44

Popular Magic Mushroom Strains _____ 48

Chapter 4: Growing Magic Mushrooms Using The PF TEK Method _____ 52

What Is The PF-Tek Approach? _____ 52

Fill The Jars With The PF Substrate _____ 56

Sterilize The PF-Tek Substrate _____ 58

Sterilizing The PF Substrate Using A Pressure Cooker _____ 61

Inoculation And Incubation Phases _____ 63

Injecting The Substrate With Spores _____ 64

Cultivation Phase _____ 69

Storing The Mushrooms _____ 74

Chapter 5: The 6 S Technique To Enhance The Effectiveness Of A Psychedelic Experience _____ 77

Set _____ 77

Setting _____ 80

*Substance*_____ 82

*Sitter*_____ 83

Session _____ 84

Situation _____ 85

Conclusion _____ **87**

Chapter 1: Magic Mushrooms 101

Currently, there are more than 10,000 known species of mushrooms in the world. If this seems like a huge number to you, understand that according to mycologists (people who study and research on fungi), this is only a mere fraction of the actual number of mushroom species in the world, many of which are undiscovered.

Out of the 10,000 confirmed and discovered mushroom species, there are about 180 kinds of hallucinogenic mushrooms that are colloquially referred to as magic mushrooms. This is a special kind of mushroom specie that has unique characteristics, benefits and even side-effects.

Let's learn more about magic mushrooms before moving forward onto its cultivation.

What Are Magic Mushrooms?

Magic mushroom is a commonly used, generic term for any kind of fungi that contains psilocybin, which is a chemical that, when you ingest, produces different psychedelic experiences as well as induces an altered and heightened state of consciousness as experienced and stated by its users.

Magic mushrooms are commonly sold in the U.S. and are found throughout Europe and North America.

Psilocybin mushrooms grow wild, but can also be cultivated. The psilocybin they contain is produced naturally and is known to be a popular and strong hallucinogenic and psychoactive compound.

According to the Substance Abuse and Mental Health Services Administrations, psilocybin is one of the most powerful and well-known psychedelics. It is also categorized as a 'Schedule I' drug, in the same category as heroin, LSD, ecstasy and marijuana, which means it carries a huge potential for misuse.

Psilocybin (4-phosphoryloxy-N, N-dimethyltryptamine) and psilocin are chemicals obtained from different specific kinds of fresh or dried hallucinogenic mushrooms that are native to South America, Mexico and the northwest and southern regions of the U.S.

Psilocybin is referred to as an 'indole-alkaloids' (tryptamine.) Both compounds have a chemical structure similar to that of LSD.' Dried magic mushrooms contain around 0.2% to about 0.4% of psilocybin and psilocin in trace amounts only. Since they have a strong impact on your central nervous system and due to their addictive effect, they are often considered 'illegal.

The following image shows the chemical structure of psilocin and psilocybin.

History Of Magic Mushrooms

The psilocybin mushrooms aka 'psilocybin shrooms' have been in use for thousands of years. They are even commonly featured in prehistoric art and culture in Mesoamerica and Europe. However, Catholic missionaries believed that hallucinogenic mushrooms were not healthy and their use went against the religious and ethical teachings. This is why they rallied against the use and stamped the magic mushrooms out of America.

That said, they were grown and used by people in various indigenous ceremonies carried out in Mexico.

In 1957, an account of two ethnomusicologists was published in the 'Life' magazine, who took part in a similar indigenous ceremony. It was later revealed in 2016 that the expedition was actually funded and organized by MK-Ultra, a project of CIA. Only a year afterwards, Albert Hoffman, a chemist of Swiss origin was successful in isolating 'psilocybin', the psychedelic compound in magic mushrooms that produced the hallucinogenic effect. He was also the first chemist to synthesize LSD, which stands for Lysergic Acid Diethylamine, a popular hallucinogenic drug that brings about effects such as altered awareness, feelings and thoughts of your surroundings. On using it, you hear or see things that may not actually exist. Its physical effects include heightened blood pressured, spike in body temperature and dilated pupils.

Psilocybin mushrooms and LSD have similar effects, which is why the usage of magic mushrooms is prohibited in many cultures and countries.

That said, the mushrooms, due to their relaxing properties are still being used and cultivated. Their usage was popularized readily during the 1960s by psychedelic gurus and researchers such as Robert Anton Wilson, Terence McKenna and Timothy Leary.

For ease of learning, we will use a lot of questions to ensure you have a comprehensive understanding of magic mushrooms.

What Are The Other Names Of Magic Mushrooms?

Magic mushrooms go by many names. They are commonly referred to as 'shrooms', 'blue meanies', 'magic truffles', 'mushies', 'agaric', 'Psilocybin mushrooms', 'amani', 'liberties', philosopher's stones', 'golden tops' and 'liberty caps.'

What Are The Uses Of Psilocybin Mushrooms?

There are many uses of magic mushrooms. In this book, we will learn just a few of the many, as we will discuss more details about the use of magic mushrooms in subsequent chapters.

Magic mushrooms are used for the following issues and goals:

- They are used to trigger and accelerate personal growth. It is believed that magic mushrooms induce a mystical experience that produces feelings of complete harmony and unison with everything around you. This creates a sense of pure sacredness and elicits feelings of pure joy and peace that transcend space and time.

- They are also used to treat cluster headaches such as migraine.

- Magic mushrooms are also known to treat different mood and emotional disorders such as anxiety and depression.

- The psilocybin mushrooms are also used to treat different addictions, including substance and alcohol abuse.

- Magic mushrooms are also effective in treating eating disorders.

- Additionally, they produce feelings of pure calmness that give you a break from the chaos around you helping you sleep, feel and perform better in everyday life.

What Do Psilocybin Mushrooms Look Like?

The magic mushrooms have slender and long stems that appear greyish or white in color topped with caps that have dark gills on their underside. They look like the conventional mushrooms in many ways. In their dried form, they are rusty brown in color with off-white isolated areas.

How Are Magic Mushrooms Used?

The magic shrooms can be consumed individually, mixed with different eatables, and can also be brewed like regular tea and consumed. They are available as fresh produce, or in dried form and can be consumed in both ways. You can also mix magic mushrooms with tobacco or cannabis and smoke them.

How Do The Magic Mushrooms Taste?

Psilocybin mushrooms have a very unpalatable and bitter taste. If you cannot bear such strong tastes, it is best you do not consume it directly and individually, and instead mix it in a drink or a food item.

What Do Magic Shrooms Do To Your Body To Bring Their Effects?

Magic mushrooms are hallucinogenic drugs, which means they make you feel, hear, see and experience sensations and experiences that may seem completely real to you, but do not actually exist. The effects of these shrooms depend on your personality and nature, as well as different environmental factors.

When you consume magic mushrooms, be it in fresh or dried form, individually or in combination with another food, the psilocybin they contain is turned into psilocin in your body. It influences the levels of serotonin in your brain, which is a mood improving hormone (chemical.) When its levels rise beyond a certain level, your perception of things becomes unusual and altered. Typically, psilocybin mushrooms are used for recreational purposes.

Mushrooms, particularly magic mushrooms, have a history of being linked to helping humans understand and discover themselves and enjoy spiritual experiences.

Many people believe that weed, mushrooms and mescaline are pure, sacred herbs that can help them attain a higher spiritual state. Others, however, use magic mushrooms to experience and enjoy a sense of connection, distorted sense of space and time, and intense euphoria.

You can also have a terrifying, unpleasant and uncomfortable experience after using the magic mushrooms. This can happen with any dosage of the mushroom. It takes around 20 to 40 minutes for the magic mushrooms to induce their effects that can last for around 6 hours with the peak effects experienced 1 to 2 hours after using them. After 6 hours, psilocin is metabolized by your body and is excreted out of your system.

The effects and dose of magic shrooms vary depending on the kind of mushroom, preparation method as well as your personal tolerance level. It is usually difficult to identify the precise species of magic mushrooms, or the hallucinogen every mushroom contains.

What Are The Common Side-Effects Of Magic Mushrooms?

The commonly experienced side-effects of magic mushrooms include frequent yawning, nausea, drowsiness, nervousness, panic, psychosis, hallucination and paranoia. That said, factors such as your age, weight, dosage of magic mushrooms, your emotional state, the surrounding environment, your history of mental and physical illnesses and your personality directly affect the extent and level of the off-shoots you can experience.

Now that you have a basic understanding of what magic mushrooms are do, let us move on to discussing their usage with different dosages along with the effects produced by every dosage quantity.

Chapter 2: Effects And Side Effects Of Magic Mushrooms

Psilocybin mushrooms have a wide range of effects and side-effects that vary according to the dose of the mushrooms you ingest. Let us look at what you should expect on having magic mushrooms in any form and according to different dosage amounts.

What Happens When You Consume Psilocybin Mushrooms?

Typically, when you consume a moderate dosage of magic shrooms, which is around 1g to 2.5g, you go through intense emotional experiences. Your ability to reflect on your thoughts heightens and you experience an altered kind of psychological functioning that takes the shape of hypnagogic experiences.

This is a transitory state lying between sleep and wakefulness. Studies that examined the brain imaging of people who used magic mushrooms showed that a regular psilocybin trip neurologically resembles that of dreaming.

You also go through perceptual changes such as synesthesia, illusions, emotional shifts as well as an altered perception of time. These effects are typically experienced after about 60 minutes of orally ingesting a single dosage of 1 to 2.5 grams of psilocybin mushrooms. You start to notice different changes in your visual perception, including halos encircling objects and lights as well as various geometric patterns when you close your eyes.

In addition, you experience a shift in your emotions and thoughts. It is common to experience a unique sense of openness in your feelings and thoughts that you otherwise avoid in your routine life. You experience a sense of delight and wonder related to your surrounding environment and the different people in your life. You may discover new things about yourself; may make startling discoveries about your feelings and aspirations that you otherwise do not understand or ignore. Moreover, you start to feel a unique and newfound harmonious connection with the universe, and feel spiritually connected to it.

Ingesting magic shrooms also brings forth a range of intense emotions inside you. These can be both seemingly positive and negative emotions such as joy, ecstasy, peace, envy and anger. Experts advise not to ignore or resist these feelings; rather embrace them as you experience them and allow them to run their full course. If you feel anger bubble inside you, let it rise and subside on its own instead of trying to control it. If you feel a surge of ecstasy, relish it rather than pushing it deep within.

It has also been observed that those who go through intense apparently negative emotions also experience a consequent sense of calmness inside them as well as detachment from their surroundings. This is particularly true if you consciously remind yourself of how these emotions are only transitory.

Psychedelic mushrooms also come with various physical effects, including a sudden spike or drop in your blood pressure, heightened tendon reflexes, dilated pupils, tremors, nausea, arousal or restlessness and experiencing trouble with different coordinated movements.

One study discovered that psilocybin usage can result in headaches that last from a few hours to a full day, even in the healthiest of individuals. The subjects reported extreme headaches. This contradicts with the finding that if used correctly, magic mushroom helps treat cluster headaches.

The different effects experienced during and after ingesting psychedelic mushrooms are known as a magic mushroom trip.' A regular psychedelic mushroom trip comprises of four phases: ingestion, onset, the peak aka trip phase and the last phase referred to as the 'comedown.' Each of these four phases come with their own set of observations and perceptions, with intense psychological and sensory shifts experienced during the peak phase that is experienced 1 to 2 hours after ingesting the magic shrooms.

You are likely to experience a bad psychedelic mushroom trip too that comprises of uncontrollable paranoia, dysphoric hallucinations and strange, reckless behaviors. You can however avoid these bad trips by following the 6S's to have a good psychedelic experience. These will be discussed in one of the following chapters.

To make the most of a magic mushroom trip, remember to relax as much as possible and wrap your head around the fact that every experience is temporary, even those that appear negative and seem to shake you. Prior to moving forward, let's discuss what a psychedelic experience is and does to you.

What Is A Psychedelic Experience?

A psychedelic experience is induced by psychedelics, chemicals that stimulate different regions of your brain that produce an altered state of awareness, realization and consciousness. These experiences are usually compared to profound meditative states, near death experiences (NDEs), out of body experiences (OBEs) and dreaming.

These experiences give you deep, immense and enlightening knowledge about your subconscious mind. A deep psychedelic experience could be very eye opening for you. It gives insight into what you want and can even help you take important decisions regarding your life. Usually, a single experience is sufficient for you to understand and transform your life.

How Magic Shrooms Interact With Different Food Items And Drugs

Magic shrooms have interesting interactions with different drugs and food items.

- **Marijuana**: You can mix psychedelic mushrooms with marijuana, as there is no known danger of creating this combination. The psychedelic experience will only enhance by this concoction.

- **Coffee**: The coffee and magic mushroom combination is often referred to as a 'cosmic stratosphere match.' The two work well together and can offer you a fantastic psychedelic experience.

- **Zoloft, Xanax and Adderall**: All the three are strong psychoactive drugs. They are also notorious for producing different side-effects. However, you can combine any of these with psychedelic mushrooms, but you need to approach the mixture with great care and use it in small quantities.

Effects Of Magic Mushrooms By Dose

The following dose ranges are for the Psilocybe cubensis mushroom specie and are applicable to the other magic mushroom species too.

Microdose (0.05-0.25 g)

- Mood enhancement

- Emotional stability

- Stress reduction

- Mindfulness, presence of mind, and peacefulness

- Increased empathy

- Sociability

- Openness

- Self-forgiveness

- Alleviation of persistent conditions such as anxiety, depression, ADD/ADHD, PTSD

- Conversational fluidity

- Increased focus and productivity

- Increased motivation

- Clearer, rational and more connected thinking

- Increased flow states

- Improved memory

- Heightened senses

- Enhanced appreciation for music, culture, art, and many others

- Spontaneity

- Increased creativity

- Easier meditation

- Relaxation and increased awareness of body

- Increased involvement and enjoyment of physical activity and routine tasks

- Enhanced athletic endurance

- Increased energy overall (without anxiety or a subsequent crash)

- Slight sedative effect

- Amplification of mood both, positive or negative

- Potentially increased neuroticism

- Possible manic states

Mini-Dose (0.25-0.75 g)

- Mood enhancement

- Mild euphoria or excitement

- Mindfulness, presence of mind, and peace

- Openness

- Self-forgiveness

- Introspective insights

- Increased motivation such as the drive to make positive lifestyle changes)

- Alleviation of persistent conditions such as depression, anxiety, ADD/ADHD, PTSD

- Increased flow states

- Clearer and rational thinking

- Enhanced appreciation for music, art, and more

- Enhanced senses

- Enhanced creativity

- Spontaneity

- Increased engagement and enjoyment of physical activity and routine tasks

- Easier meditation

- Relaxation and increased awareness of body

- Mild body high

- Increased energy in waves

- Amplification of mood both, positive or negative

- Increased sensitivity to light

- Preference for introspection over socializing

- Very mild visuals, if any

- Potentially increased neuroticism

- Possible manic states

- Difficulty focusing or thought loops

- Anxiety, agitation and restlessness

- Difficulty with some cognitive tasks

- Difficulty or discomfort socializing

- Frustration at dosage (too high to be comfortable, too low to be "recreational")

Museum Dose (0.5-1.5 g)

- Mild to moderate visuals (e.g. "breathing" environments)

- Mood enhancement, euphoria or excitement

- Increased empathy

- Introspection

- Conversational fluidity

- Enhanced senses

- Increased flow states

- Enhanced appreciation for music, culture and art, and more

- Enhanced creativity

- Spontaneity

- Finding otherwise routine things hilarious or interesting

- Enhanced athletic endurance

- Increased enjoyment of physical activity and routine tasks

- Moderate body high

- Clear come-up, peak, and come-down

- Stimulation and amplification of mood both, positive or negative

- Altered perception of sound

- Increased sensitivity to light

- Time dilation or contraction (time passing more slowly or quickly)

- Pupil dilation

- Difficulty with some tasks

- Difficulty focusing

- Difficulty or discomfort socializing

- Frustration at dosage (at lower end)

Moderate Dose (2-3.5 g)

- Sense of peacefulness and relaxation

- Strong euphoria or excitement

- Mystical experience and feelings of wonder

- Increased flow of creative and unique ideas

- Life-changing introspective or philosophical insights

- Heightened creativity

- Enhanced appreciation for music

- Heightened senses

- Strong body high

- Finding otherwise routine and boring things funny or interesting

The Complete Psilocybin Mushroom Blueprint

- Clear come-up, peak, and come-down

- Open- and closed-eye visuals (e.g. patterns, auras)

- Amplification of emotions, whether good or bad

- Synesthesia

- Sedation

- Feeling of time passing more slowly or quickly

- Unusual physical sensations

- Wide pupil dilation

- Sensitivity to light

- Compulsive yawning

- Disorientation

- Confusion

- Difficulty with cognitive tasks

- Fear and anxiety

- Nausea

- Dizziness

Mega Dose (5+ g)

- Mystical experience and intense feelings of wonder

- Strong euphoria or excitement

- Ego death

- Heightened creativity

- Life-changing introspective or philosophical insights

- Enhanced senses

- Increased flow of ideas

- Very strong body high

- Finding seemingly mundane situations or experiences interesting/funny

- Clear come-up followed by a peak, and then instant come-down

- You feel your memories coming to life

- Amplification of different good and bad emotions

- Very strong open- and closed-eye visions

- Visual, auditory, tactile hallucinations

- Synesthesia

- Increased thought loops

- Time becoming meaningless

- Sedation

- Sensitivity to light

- Very wide pupil dilation

- Unusual physical sensations and altered perception of physical form

- Confusion

- Compulsive yawning

- Disorientation

- Strong fear and anxiety (extreme "bad trip" experiences)

- Compromised motor functions (sitter recommended!)

- Extreme difficulty with cognitive tasks

- Nausea

- Dizziness

- Headaches

- Light-headedness

Benefits Of Psychedelic Mushrooms

Many studies are being carried out on psychedelic mushrooms and how they influence the human body and mind. One particular study published in the 'Journal of Psychopharmacology' illustrates that only one dose of magic shrooms produces an enduring and substantial reduction in anxiety and depression, and improves the quality of your life.

The many profound and mystical psychedelic mushrooms are believed to produce effects that have been felt and enjoyed by many people since the 1960s. This is what compelled the researchers and scientists to delve deeper into the matter and figure out the actual effects of magic mushrooms on the human mind, body and spirit.

Many clinical trials have so far been conducted on the subjects who use psilocybin mushrooms. These trials help understand how different doses of these mushrooms administered to the subjects in a therapeutic environment reduce their anxiety and stress, particularly the stress that comes from being diagnosed with life-threatening conditions such as cancer.

So far, the results have been very promising. In double-lined conditions, a single, high dose of magic mushrooms has demonstrated a good reduction in psychological stress in patients suffering from terminal health conditions.

Let us look on the different effects and benefits of psilocybin mushrooms on different aspects of your health and wellbeing.

Personal Growth

During the early trials, psychedelic mushrooms were administered to healthy adults in well-monitored and supportive conditions. It was observed that the majority of the participants experienced long lasting positive improvements in their values, behaviors, attitudes and personality.

The subjects reported a higher appreciation and enjoyment of art, culture, music and nature. Moreover, they experienced a higher tolerance level along with increased creative abilities. They were able to think better and creatively that enabled them to put a positive spin on the difficult situations they encountered in life.

Recently conducted studies on the subject have mirrored these findings as well. A whopping 40% of the participants of these laboratory studies exhibited a very positive change in their attitude towards life, relationship with nature and their aesthetic sense. A study conducted in 2011 discovered that even after a year of having a single experience with magic shrooms, the subjects continued to live positively and had a very open and welcoming approach towards life. Researchers also speculate that the mystical experience produced by these mushrooms is the reason behind such enduring and positive changes.

The mystical experience is defined as feeling united with everything around them that brings forth a sense of peace, sacredness and harmony. It has also been observed that those who report more intense mystical experiences benefit from the positive changes for a long time.

This feeling of interconnectedness brought about by the psilocybin mushrooms is due to the reduction in the interconnectedness of the many integration regions in your brain. Psilocybin enables for a better cross talk between the different brain hubs that are otherwise kept separate. When you consume a single dose of magic shrooms, the different regions of your brain begin to operate as one and have a higher connectivity with each other. This brings about a state of complete 'unconstrained cognition' that allows you to feel and think better and freely. These effects are similar to those brought about by deep meditation.

Recently conducted research studies on the topic have shown that psilocybin mushrooms can be used to improve your spiritual connection with yourself as well.

A huge study conducted on 75 participants engaged them in a spiritual course spanning over six months. It comprised of activities centered on introspection, awareness, mindfulness and meditation. During the six month program, the participants were also administered either a high or a low dose of the psychedelic mushrooms. After the course was over, the participants who were administered high doses of psilocybin mushrooms showed a higher improvement in their spirituality levels such as closeness with themselves and a better understanding of death, life purpose in life, forgiveness and transcendence as compared to those who were given a low dose of these mushrooms.

Soothes And Cures Cluster Headaches

Numerous preclinical trials conducted during the 1960s and 1970s suggested that psychedelic mushrooms had a promising role in treating cluster headaches, addiction and mood disorders.

Researchers on the subject became non-existent after the psychedelic mushrooms were termed as 'Schedule I drug' by the federal government in the late 1970s. However, research is now being conducted on magic mushrooms by organizations like The John Hopkins Center for Psychedelic & Consciousness Research, MAPS and The Beckley Foundation.

Cluster headaches are similar to migraines, with the difference being that the former are shorter in duration and more intense as compared to the latter. They are described as the most disruptive and painful headaches that exist by those who suffer from them. Attacks during the night tend to be more painful as compared to those endured in the daytime, but both attacks significantly interfere with your life.

While there are no systematic research studies conducted on the effects of psychedelic mushrooms on reducing cluster headaches, there are scores of anecdotal reports to prove that.

During the mid-2000s, researchers and doctors took notice of the effect of psychedelics on cluster headaches when some patients suffering from the headaches reported to experience a significant improvement in them. Different surveys were then conducted on the subject matter.

A recently conducted survey on the topic reports that magic mushrooms are indeed very effective in treating cluster headaches as compared to the currently available medicines for the problem. Around 50% of people who experience cluster headaches report a massive improvement in the intensity and duration of their headaches.

Helps Relieve Anxiety And Mood Disorders

Different anecdotal evidence points towards the remarkable positive effects of psychedelic mushrooms in relieving anxiety, stress and mood disorders. Dr. James Fadiman is a pioneer researcher in the area who has been gathering anecdotes relevant to the subject for years.

The federal government has allowed the conduction of a few, highly controlled studies on the matter that has proven that psychedelic mushrooms indeed have a therapeutic effect on mood disorders. In 2011, a pilot study was carried out to test the different effects of psilocybin mushrooms on anxiety and depression in patients suffering from cancer.

Patients in this particular study suffered from advanced-stage of cancer along with anxiety and stress that stemmed from the diagnosis of their cancer. The researchers found out that after consuming psilocybin mushrooms, the patients experienced a reduction in their anxiety and depression for up to six months.

A religious research group working in London conducted a study that illustrated how psychedelic mushrooms were effective in treating depression. Twelve patients suffering from depression were divided into two groups: one was given a high dose of magic mushrooms whereas the other was administered a low dose of the same. A week after receiving the dose, depression scores of all the patients had dropped low, and 8 out of 12 patients exhibited no signs and symptoms of depression at all. About three months after the treatment, 5 of 12 patients remained free of depression and 4 of the remaining 7 saw their depression reduce from severe to mild.

The psilocybin mushroom treatment has also been proven to be successful in reducing the symptoms of obsessive-compulsive disorder (OCD) in a study conducted on patients suffering from the problem. The patients did not respond positively to serotonin reuptake inhibitor (SRI) drug therapy, but showed a massive reduction in their OCD levels after going through the psychedelic mushroom therapy.

Helps Treat Addictions

Psychedelic mushrooms were also used in preclinical trials to cure addiction during the 1950s and 1960s. All the trials illustrated promising results and helped people suffering from alcohol and drug abuse slowly overcome their addictive behaviors. However, when the magic shrooms were made illegal in the majority of Europe and U.S., the research studies conducted on the topic dropped low too.

However, there has been resurgence in the use of psychedelic mushrooms to treat addictions in recent years. In 2015, a study conducted on the subject showed that magic shrooms were indeed very effective in overcoming alcohol addiction. Reductions in the extent of drinking as well as abstinence were reported by the participants of the study after going through a psilocybin mushroom treatment.

It has also been observed that magic mushrooms are helpful in helping one quit smoking and tobacco abuse. A recently conducted trial on the subject showed those who had 2 to 3 psilocybin mushroom treatment sessions experienced a 80% success rate in quitting smoking. On the other hand, other methods to quit smoking such as quitting cold turkey, chewing gum and using nicotine patches have only a 35% success rate. This proves that psilocybin mushrooms are indeed a more effective and promising treatment approach to quitting smoking for good.

The different effects of psychedelic mushrooms in helping you overcome mood disorders, addictions, obsessive compulsive disorders and experiencing an improvement in the quality of life are related to their ability to rewire your brain. The DMN (default mode network) center in your brain is associated with the onset of depression, mood disorders and addictions. Psilocybin mushrooms reset this control system and reduce the DMN's activity. This helps you calm down and take better control of yourself.

Now that you have a better knowledge of how beneficial magic mushrooms are, let us move our focus to cultivation.

Chapter 3: Growing Magic Mushrooms With Ready To Use Kits

One great quality about growing magic mushrooms is that there are various ways to do that. You can choose a method that best suits your style. There are many psychedelic mushroom grow Teks (techniques) floating around and from this chapter onwards, we will discuss them. Arguably, the most commonly used and popular mushroom grow tek is the PF Tek that will be discussed separately in the next chapter.

The easiest and simplest way to cultivate magic shrooms is through a ready to grow kit or a mycelium box. These are pre-made mushroom growing kits that come with a substrate, mycelium of a specie of the psilocybin mushroom and a casing layer.

Psilocybin Mushroom Ready To Grow Kit With Substrate

A magic shroom substrate kit comes with a pre-sterilized substrate made of grass-sed, white rice, brown rice, vermiculite flour or rye. There can be other combinations too, but mostly, these ingredients are used.

All you need to do is add your own spores to the substrate and your magic mushrooms will grow in no time. This method usually takes a few weeks to have fully grown magic mushrooms.

If you don't already know, understand that mushroom substrate refers to the bulk material that serves as the major food source by the mushroom mycelium. Commonly used substrates include baled grasses, hay, cereal straw, sawdust, used coffee grounds, paper, coffee waste, coniferous trees, sugarcane bagasse and wood shavings.

The rule of thumb for use of wood substrates such as sawdust and shavings is to take wood from any hardwood tree species with broad leaves. Avoid using sawdust from aromatic or coniferous trees. Make sure the mushroom substrate you use is properly prepared. Add enough supplements to it and provide it with enough moisture. You would also need to effectively sterilize it so it becomes ready to colonize the chosen magic shroom strain. In optimal conditions, your shroom mycelium will colonize the substrate and produce mushrooms in a few weeks.

Growing Magic Shrooms Using Mushroom Spawn Bags

A mushroom spawn bag usually refers to two things. Some people refer to it as a grow bag that contains a substrate. On the other hand, certain people refer to a bag containing a mycelium-colonized substrate as a spawn bag. It has a substrate that is inoculated with any mushroom strain that is fully colonized. It is known as a spawn, and from this spawn, you can inoculate a large amount of substrate.

To make a mushroom spawn, you need to have a sterile environment. First, you need spores from any magic mushroom strain you want to grow. You also need substrate such as straw, wood chips or white rice. Make sure to sterilize the substrate and then inoculate it with the spores you have chosen.

Here are the steps you can follow to grow your mushroom strain in a rye or spawn bag.

- You can easily find a spawn bag from brick and mortar stores or on e-stores.

- Every bag comes with a self-healing injector site that closes once you pull its needle out.

- The white square filter patch is located towards the bag's top. It allows complete gas exchange to grow the strain, but also filters the contaminants.

- Prior to starting the cultivation, ensure that you inject the spore in the bag in a clean environment. It is best to use a sterile spore injection for the purpose.

- You need to wipe the syringe clean as well as the black spot- the injection site with a clean, alcohol swab.

- Pull the syringe needle's cover away from your syringe.

- Flame the syringe's needle until it becomes piping hot.

- Wait for about 3 to 5 seconds for it to cool down a little.

- Once it is slightly cooler than before, push in the needle around ½ inches into the spawn bag.

- Inject around 2 to 3 cc's of the mushroom spores.

- It is recommended you use a total of around 4 to 5 cc's of the mushroom spores per spawn bag.

- Ensure to inject the spores in several locations in the spawn bag so it spreads well in the bag.

- Unroll your spawn bag and enure the filter patch is completely upright.

- Very gently, pull its two sides apart and be cautious in not touching the white part of the filter. Your goal should be to create a path right from the grain towards the filter.

- Gently place the spawn bag in a dark, warm location. The temperature should be around 75 to 77 degrees optimally.

- Leave the spawn bags to incubate.

- Spawn bags colonize from their inside out unlike the jars so you will not see any mushroom growth for about two weeks.

- Spawn bags produce their own heat internally while they colonize so the inside temperature of the inside of a spawn bag is about 3 to 4 degrees warmer than the outside temperature.

- After about 14 days, you will notice white colored mycelium slowly growing and spreading inside the spawn bag.

- Spawn bags are well known for completely colonizing on their own without doing anything special except for maintaining their temperature.

- When the spawn bags colonize about 20 to 30%, or when it has been about 18 days since you placed spores in them, try a technique to increase the growth speed of the strains. Use your fingers to knead the bag so you break up the white mycelium into tiny pieces. Make sure you do not puncture the bag with your nails.

- Once the white mycelium is well spread around the bag, repack the grain into its original shape.

- Grab the bag from the top and drop it on a counter.

- Practice this step a couple of times.

- This packs the grains back down.

- If you notice any loose grain, press it using your fingers and ensure there are no spaces or air gaps in the bag.

- Now place the bag in the incubation chamber again and do not disturb it at least for 4 weeks.

- You will not observe any progress in a few days, but after 10 days, you will notice good growth all across the bag.

- This progress will carry on until the spawn bag is 100% colonized.

- Full colonization will take around 30 to about 45 days, depending on the type of magic mushroom strain you have chosen and the temperature of the incubation chamber.

This is an easy technique for beginners. However, for any technique, you need to choose a mushroom strain.

Popular Magic Mushroom Strains

Here are 5 of the most popular magic shroom strains you can use to grow your own magic mushrooms at home.

1. B+ Psilocybe Cubensis Strain

This is a great strain for beginners who are not yet used to growing magic mushrooms. This strain has the ability to easily adjust to different temperatures, substrates and conditions and grow successfully. Legend holds that a very dedicated cultivator known as 'Mr G.' from Florida created this strain in the 90s. The strain then completely took the psychedelic mushroom community by storm and has since then been referred to as the 'best mushroom strain.'

The B+ strain is a huge growing cubensis strain that can quickly grow into a huge fungi. Since it is adaptable with all weather conditions, it is best to start off your mushroom cultivation journey with this amazing strain.

2. PES Amaonian Psilocybe Cubensis Strain

If you are in search of an authentic, one of a kind psychedelic experience, it is recommended you try the PES Amazonian strain, particularly if you want instant relief from the stress and anxiety you have been going through for a long time. Pacifica Spora, a company that discovered this strain in the Amazonian jungle, created this strain.

With this strain, you can expect fleshy, big magic shrooms having a height of more than 6 inches on average, with some mushrooms reaching about 12 inches.

3. McKennaii Psilocybe Cubensis Strain

This strain is perfect for those who take magic mushroom cultivation seriously. This self-resilient strain grows well in different conditions and provides users with a mesmerizing, profound psychedelic experience.

With a high dose, you will transcend into another world and have a truly enchanting experience. If you have just ventured into the magic mushroom experience, it is best to start with the B+ strain and later opt for the McKennaii strain once you have grown and used the B+ strain a few times.

4. Golden Teacher Psilocybe Cubensis Strain

This strain is an absolute favorite amongst the avid magic mushroom cultivators. It is loved because it grows great flushes and provides a truly amazing psychedelic journey.

This strain does not bear spres fast as the other strains discussed above, as it grows in less than optimal conditions, but since it can grow in harsh weather conditions, mushroom growers love it. If you want to have a deep self-reflection experience and tap into your spirituality, the Golden Teacher is the perfect strain for you.

5. Mazatapec Psilocybe Cubensis Strain

The Mazatapec magic shrooms are rich with the wildlife of Middle America and grow into large flushes with luxurious brown caps. You just need to be patient while growing this strain as it has an old, mystical soul that takes more than a few weeks to grow. However, this strain results in brilliant magic shrooms that can help you unlock great wisdom and spirituality.

It is a wise move to start with the first strain and once you have enjoyed a few psychedelic experiences; you can choose the more mature strains and deepen your psychedelic experiences.

Chapter 4: Growing Magic Mushrooms Using The PF TEK Method

PF-Tek is a very easy approach for cultivating magic shrooms. Its biggest benefit is that all the materials and supplies required are easy to find and the substrate can easily be prepared using household items. Let me give you better insight into the method so you can easily follow it at home.

What Is The PF-Tek Approach?

PF is short form for Psylocybe Fanaticus while Tek is short form for technique. Robert Billy McPherson came up with the approach.

Its substrate proved to be the optimal soil for psilocybe cubensis shrooms. The PF-original spores are named after Mr. Fanaticus. The PF Tek manual is now being followed by mushroom growers across the globe primarily because it is incredibly simple to follow and helps ordinary people create substrate cakes in no time.

PF Tek helps cultivators in growing magic shrooms from scratch, is affordable, easy to follow and comes with a high success rate.

List Of Supplies And Materials

To grow mushrooms using the PF Tek technique, you need the following items and materials.

Substrate

- Water

- Vermiculite

- Brown rice flour

Supplies

- Covers

- Jars

- Aluminum foil

- Grow bag

- Regular pan or pressure cooker

- Spore syringe, spore print or spore vial

- Torch lighter or alcohol burner

- Syringe

- Gloves

- Respirator/ face mask

- Mixing bowl

- Measuring cup

- Scale

- Spoon/ fork

- Marker

- Labels or tape

- Drill, awl, nail and hammer

Making The PF- Tek Substrate

Here is how you can create the PF-Tek substrate:

Make sure to mix in the substrate ingredients in the exact ratio mentioned below to prepare the ideal soil to cultivate your magic mushrooms. The ratio you should use is 2:1:1, i.e. two parts of vermiculite, one part of brown rice flour and one part of water.

The following table shows the quantities of these three ingredients that you should use depending on the size and number of the jars you are using.

Jar 240ml (½ pint)	Vermiculite	Brown rice flour	Water
1 jar	120 ml	60 ml	60 ml
4 jars	480 ml	240 ml	240 ml
6 jars	720 ml	360 ml	360 ml
8 jars	960 ml	480 ml	480 ml

When you mix the PF-Tek substrate, make sure to use a bowl that is big enough to hold all the ingredients. Using a small bowl will only result in spillage and waste of materials. Also, clean the bowl thoroughly and sterilize it if possible before adding the ingredients to it for mixing.

- First, spread vermiculite in the bowl.

- Slowly add in some water and mix it well with the substrate. Gradual addition of water is crucial so you do not make the substrate too wet and soggy. The water amount will have to be adjusted according to the quality and quantity of brown rice four and vermiculite being used as the higher the quality of the brown rice flour and vermiculite the more the water they absorb. Never add all the water in one go to the PF substrate.

- The substrate needs to be damp enough to moisturize the strains, but should not be soaked.

- Hold the bowl by tilting on its side so no water pours out.

- Now add in the brown rice flour.

- Mix in the ingredients thoroughly.

Once you have followed all these steps, your PF-Tek substrate is ready to be used.

Fill The Jars With The PF Substrate

Next, you need to fill in your jars with the substrate you have prepared. For this phase, you need substrate, spoon/ fork, vermiculite, aluminum foil or covers, awl and alcohol wipe.

Here is what you need to do next.

- Take the fork and use it to gently loosen up the PF substrate.

- Ensure that the substrate mix does not contain any big chunks.

- Next, top it with a layer of vermiculite. The vermiculite serves as a filter layer between the air and the PF substrate, keeping out all the microorganisms that may contaminate your PF-Tek.

- Gently and thoroughly clean the jar's edge using alcohol wipe. If an alcohol wipe isn't available, kitchen paper would work fine too.

- Place aluminum foil or a lid/ cover on the jar to cover it tightly. It is wise to have both ready before you begin filling in the jars.

- Practice the same steps with all the jars that you are using to grow mushrooms.

- Shake your substrate gently so it spreads in the jar evenly. Make sure the substrate is airy enough so that all the spores and then the mycelium spread in it easily.

Here is how you can prepare a cover or an aluminum foil to cover the jar.

- Cover: Take the drill or awl to puncture five holes in the cover that will later help you spray the spores inside the jar. Create four holes in every corner of the cover's edge and one hole right in the center. You can create holes with the help of a hammer and nail as well.

- Aluminum Foil: Cut out three strokes of about 15 centimeters each per jar. The foil you use must be big enough to completely cover the jar's top side. Take two layers of the foil to completely cover the jar, as this is the point that you will pierce through using the spore syringe. Just ensure that the part can be taken off easily.

Once you have prepared the two, use either to cover the jar. When the jar is prepared, you need to sterilize the PF-Tek substrate.

Sterilize The PF-Tek Substrate

For this stage, you need jars containing the substrate, a high pan with a lid or a pressure cooker, water, foil/ covers, cooking counter, heat source/ gas cooker, marker and tape. This is a crucial step, as you need to effectively sterilize the substrate to kill off any contaminants that may be in it such as microorganisms and bacteria. You can sterilize the jar using either of the two ways: using a regular pan covered with a lid or with a pressure cooker. Both approaches will sterilize your substrate through steam.

Let us discuss both these methods one by one.

Sterilizing The PF Substrate In A Regular Pan

- Take a big sized, deep enough pan with a tight cover that can easily accommodate everything.

- Place a rack at the bottom of the pan. You can even use covers for this purpose. This prevents the jars from coming into contact with the pan's hot bottom and keep them from shattering.

- Open the substrate jar's cover slightly, and use foil to cover it.

- Place all the PF substrate jars in the frying pan.

- Fill in the pan with water to about 1 centimeter underneath the jars' edge.

- Place the pan on the heat source and very slowly start to heat the pan.

- Bring the water in the pan to boil.

- Let it simmer and steam for about 90 minutes. Make sure you have covered the pan with a lid.

- Keep the flame as low as possible so the water in the pan continues to boil and steam.

- Every few minutes, take a peek at the pan to ensure it has sufficient water in it.

- After 90 minutes, turn off the heat. You can let it steam for long to completely sterilize the substrate, but then you would have to observe extra caution to ensure the water doesn't dry out and check the pan frequently.

- When you have turned off the heat, leave the jars in the frying pan to cool off. This can take up one whole night, but at the minimum, it takes about 5 hours.

- When the jars have cooled down, take them out of the pan, one by one and label each of the jars with a letter, number, symbol or anything else so you can discern among them easily.

Your jars are now all set to be inoculated with the magic mushroom spores.

Sterilizing The PF Substrate Using A Pressure Cooker

- Go through your pressure cooker's manual and try it out with another food item first prior to sterilizing your PF substrate jars in it. This helps you identify any faults or issues in it, and fix them beforehand.

- Once you are ready to use your pressure cooker, place a rack or covers on the bottom of the cooker to ensure the jars do not come into direct contact with the hot cooker and do not crack.

- Pour in water to fill in the pressure cooker to about 4 to 5 centimeters from the bottom. You can also do it as mentioned in its manual.

- Place all the PF substrate jars on the covers or rack in the cooker.

- Close the cooker with its lid.

- Place the cooker on the stove and switch on the heating source.

- Keep the flame on low heat so the cooker gently heats and reaches the right pressure, which is mostly one atmosphere or 15 psi.

- Let the cooker steam for about 45 to 60 minutes.

- After an hour, turn off the heat.

- Allow the jars in the pressure cooker to cool off which takes around 5 to 11 hours.

- When the jars are cool, take them out of the pressure cooker and label them like taught before so you can easily tell every jar apart.

Your PF substrate jars are ready to be inoculated with your chosen mushroom strain. Be sure to smell your PF substrate prior to sterilizing it, and then after you have sterilized it. This helps you figure out the difference in its smell before or after the sterilization. If the smell is too pungent and sour, it may be indicative of a contamination that has taken place in the jar.

Keep all the PF-substrate jars for one whole week at room temperature in a draft-free and dark place. Check all the jars after a week for any contaminations by smelling them to ensure you do not inoculate contaminated jars with your mushroom spores. If any jar is contaminated, get rid of it to prevent the contaminants from spreading to other jars. Disinfect the entire area before placing other jars in it.

Inoculation And Incubation Phases

For these phases, you need your mushroom spores, sterilized substrate jars, spray, foil, alcohol burner or a lighter, facemask, gloves and a disinfecting gel. Inoculating the PEF-Tek substrate is the second most important phase of the method. You need to work cautiously in a sterile environment.

Be sure to properly clean the space you are working in prior to injecting your substrate jars with the mushroom spores. You need to sanitize your hands with a disinfecting gel and a respirator prior to starting the process. Moreover, creating an inoculation space or a glove box are wise moves too, but it is not a mandatory step.

To inoculate the jars, use a syringe to inject the spores to your substrate that you prepared earlier. The mushroom spores will develop into mycelium that will gradually colonize the entire substrate in the jar.

You need at least a 1ml spore solution to colonize one jar. You can use a 2ml solution too if you want to colonize the substrate cake faster. The spore sprayers usually available contain about 10 to 20ml spore solution that is sufficient to colonize about 10 to 20 of the substrate jars you have been taught to prepare.

Injecting The Substrate With Spores

You then need to inject the jars with your mushroom strain spores. Here is a step by step procedure to do that cautiously and successfully.

- Check all the jars thoroughly for any contamination by smelling them.

- Disinfect the entire workspace.

- Wash your hands thoroughly and then put on the respirator. Gloves are optional, but definitely a good safety measure.

- Prepare all the things you need such as spore syringe, foil, jars and burner.

- Prepare your spore syringe as mentioned on the instructions that come with it.

- Heat the syringe's needle until it becomes red hot.

- Let it cool for a few seconds.

- Take the foil off from the cover. If you are only using the foil, remove only its top layer.

- Stick in the spore syringe's needle throughout the foil or cover right along the jar's edge.

- Press the syringe gently until one drop of the spore solution sprinkles out.

- Very slowly, move the syringe's needle upwards, taking it out of the substrate jar while you press the sprayer. This makes the spores easily spread all across the jar's edge.

- Heat the syringe's needle until it becomes red hot after you inject it in the jar every time. However, wait for a few seconds to let it cool down prior to injecting it another time.

- Be sure to inject it in the jar on at least four spots near its edge and at least one in the center too.

- 1 ml of the spore solution is good enough to colonize the entire jar.

- Once you have inoculated it, tightly cover the jar with foil.

- Repeat the steps for all the substrate jars.

- Ensure to write the date of the inoculation on every jar along with the spray you have used to tell them apart. This way, you can compare the psychedelic experience brought about by the different strains and find out the ones that work best for you.

Once you have injected all the substrate jars with your mushroom spores, you need to wait for some time so the mycelium completely colonizes every jar.

Make sure to place the jars in a draft-free and dark place. The temperature of the space needs to be around 27 degrees Celsius. The jars will not colonize if the temperature drops below 15 degrees Celsius so take care in that regard.

The complete colonization of the entire PF-Tek substrate jar can take around 4 weeks depending on the surrounding environment's conditions. After 3 to 7 days of inoculating the substrates, you will observe the early signs of mycelium formation. This is recognized by the pearly white threads that start to grow out from all the spots you injected the mushroom spores in. Once the entire jar is white, wait for another week so the inside of the PF-Tek substrate is completely colonized too.

You need to observe the PF-Tek substrate jars throughout the incubation phase for any contaminations. If a contamination has started, the growing mycelium will take on a different hue. Healthy mycelium is white, but if it gets contaminated, it can take on a greenish, orang-ish, velvety, blackish, grayish or a yellowish hue.

The moment you discover that a jar is contaminated, quickly discard the substrate. Thoroughly wash your hands and then disinfect the entire workspace as well as the incubation environment of the substrate jars. You need to ensure the contamination does not spread to the other healthy substrate jars. Take note on the jars that became contaminated, the color they changed, the number of days after which the contamination appears, how the contamination appeared and the probable cause of the contamination.

Once the entire substrate has been colonized by the mycelium, the chance of a contamination is quite bleak. The mycelium is a living organism and has the potential to fight off many contaminations itself as it tries its best to survive and grow.

For the cultivation phase, you can also prepare a growing chamber.

To make a shotgun fruiting chamber, here is what you should do.

- Take a plastic storage container.

- Drill ¼ inch holes in it about 2 inches away all across the lid, base and sides.

- Drill the holes right from the container's inside out on to a block of wood to make sure the container does not crack.

- Set the box on four stable items, arranged right at the corners so air flows underneath it.

- You can cover the surface underneath the box to keep it safe from moisture leakage.

- You can place the perlite in a strainer and let cold water run over it to soak it.

- Let the water drain so there are no drips at all.

- Spread the soaked perlite over the cultivation chamber.

- Repeat for another layer of perlite around 4 to 5 inches deep.

This is an easy and quick method to create a fruiting chamber that works well for novices.

Cultivation Phase

For this phase, you need the colonized PF-Tek substrate jars, cover, fork or spoon, paper clip, cultivation bag, gloves, plant sprayer, respirator, disinfectant solution and vermiculite or perlite (these are optional though.)

If your substrate has grown fully after four weeks and is not contaminated, you are ready to proceed to the final step of the process: preparing your substrate cakes to grow your magic mushrooms. To start growing your magic shrooms, you will have to take out the substrate cakes from the jar.

Here is a step by step process of the cultivation phase.

- Open the substrate's cover. If you have covered it using a foil, take off that.

- Very carefully, remove the vermiculite lying on the cake's top. Use a sterile fork to do that.

- You are likely to find mycelium here. Remove it together with the vermiculite.

- Take a plate or cover that is slightly large as compared to the PF-Tek's substrate jar and place it on the jar.

- Place the jar upside down.

- Very gently, tap the PF-Tek substrate loose.

- Now allow the substrate to gently glide out of the jar so it rests on the plate or cover you are using.

- Place the PF-Tek substrate cake on the cover right in the cultivation bag. There is likely to be enough room for two cakes in a single cultivation bag, but if there isn't, use one cake per bag.

- Sprinkle some water in the cultivation bag with the help of the plant sprayer so it has the right humidity level.

- Repeat these steps for all the PF-Tek substrate cakes to cultivate your mushrooms.

Wait for another 1 to 2 weeks and you will have lovely mushrooms at your disposal.

The Complete Psilocybin Mushroom Blueprint

For best mushroom growth, ensure to take care of the following:

- The optimal cultivation environment temperature for the magic mushroom strains is 24 degrees Celsius.

- The humidity level in the cultivation bag with the mycelium must be 95%.

- The air in the bag needs to be refreshed before you close it again. It must have a good amount of oxygen and a little carbon dioxide. To keep the air appropriately humid and moist, cover the jar with a nice layer of burlap. This enables the air to properly circulate through to the strain, and traps sufficient amount of the moisture to produce a successful yield of mushrooms.

- Water the strains whenever you feel the cake becomes powdery. However, never water it straight from the faucet. Allow the water to reach room temperature in a bowl and then sprinkle it on the substrate.

- You need to provide the cultivation bags with light, but never keep them in direct sunlight.

Once the mushrooms start to appear, you need to harvest them. Remember to harvest all the mushrooms, even the tiniest of the lot. After the first flush phase, you will need to soak in the substrate cakes again for the second flush. This helps the substrate cakes get adequate moisture to produce a new flush of ripe mushrooms.

- Grab a clean bowl with clean drinking water, or a bucket containing the same.

- Place the PF-Tek substrate cake in the clean water.

- Ensure it stays deep under the water.

- Allow the cake to soak for a minimum of 12 hours.

- Take out the cake off the bucket and then place it in the cultivation bag.

- You can easily harvest 3 to 4 flushes of the magic mushrooms using the same substrate cake.

- After every harvest, remove the mushrooms and repeat the above steps.

Besides this, you can also take out the cake from the jar, soak it in water and then roll in the vermiculite. Many mycologists believe that this technique produces a better yield of magic mushrooms as the vermiculite enables the moisture to gradually dispose. This technique is referred to as the 'dunk and roll' method and can be carried out in the following manner.

- Get a clean bucket and fill it with clean drinking water.

- Place the PF-Tek substrate cakes in the bucket and ensure they stay submerged in the water.

- Let them soak for up to 12 hours.

- Get a clean plate.

- Sprinkle some vermiculite on the plate.

- Take the substrate cake out of the bucket.

- Roll the cake through the vermiculite spread on the plate.

- Repeat these steps with every substrate cake.

- Make sure to roll the cakes through the vermiculite when you prepare for the first flush. Once the first flush is over, the soaking of the cake will be quite enough for the next round of mushrooms so rolling them in the vermiculite will not be needed then.

In case you are using several PF-Tek substrate jars, try experimenting with both the methods. Half the jars can be harvested using the dunk and roll method, and half of them can be done using the previous technique. This helps you get two varieties of flushes using two different techniques so you can compare the two and find out the one that works well for you. Do mark the jars with the technique you have used.

It takes about 1 to 2 months for the mycelium colonized substrates to produce harvestable mushrooms. However, the time the mycelium takes to turn into fruit depends on several factors such as weather conditions, temperature, humidity, air quality etc. you can harvest the mushrooms about 5 to 12 days after you begin to seem them sprout from the PEF-Tek substrate.

Storing The Mushrooms

The magic mushrooms have a tendency of going bad easily if you don't store them well (storing in the fridge anyhow will make them go bad). If you want to keep them for micro-dosing or want to save them for later use, you have to be particular about their storage.

Arguably, the most effective method to store psilocybin mushrooms is to dry them up. This helps them stay potent for up to 3 years if you store them in a dry, cool and dark place. If you store them in the freezer after drying them, they will last for a good duration. However, if you store them in the fridge as they are, they will go bad within 3 to 4 weeks.

The lo-fi technique to dry the magic mushrooms is to let them rest on a sheet of dry paper for a couple of days, preferably with a fan switched on above them. The only problem with this technique is that they will not become 'cracker dry.' This means that the mushrooms will not snap when you bend them. This means they will have some moisture in them that can make them go bad after a few months.

They are likely to diminish in terms of potency too, depending on the period you leave the mushrooms out for. You can use a dehydrator to dry them as it is as incredibly effective method, albeit an expensive one.

Another potent substitute approach to dry the mushrooms is to try a dessicant.

- Air dry the magic mushrooms for about 48 hours with a fan switched on above them.

- Put a layer of the chosen dessicant on the base of a good quality, airtight container.

- The dessicants that are readily available usually include anhydrous calcium chloride and silica gel kitty litter that can be purchased easily from the hardware stores.

- Put a wire rack or something similar right over the dessicant to make sure it does not touch the mushrooms.

- Arrange the shrooms on the rack gently making certain they do not touch each other or the rack.

- Tightly seal the container.

- Wait for a week and then check the mushrooms to see if they have become cracker dry.

- Transfer the mushrooms to good quality storage bags such as vacuum-sealed or ZipLoc bags and store them in the freezer.

Use these tips and tricks, and you will keep your psilocybin mushrooms fresh for use for a couple of years.

To make the most of every psychedelic experience you have using a magic mushroom, implement the 6S technique. The next chapter walks you through it in detail.

Chapter 5: The 6 S Technique To Enhance The Effectiveness Of A Psychedelic Experience

If you are familiar with LSD use, it is likely that you may have heard the expression 'set and setting.' The term was coined by Norman Zinberg to illustrate the content for any psychedelic drug experience. Along with these two S's, you need to take care of the other 4 S's to have an amazing psychedelic experience using magic mushrooms.

The 6 S's in the 6 S approach stand for: set, setting, substance, sitter, session and situation. The primary role is played by 'set' and 'setting', but the other 4 S's, if observed correctly, do improve the experience too.

Set

Set stands for the 'mindset' you observe while taking a psychedelic trip. It comprises of the preparation of the voyager (you in case you are going on a magic mushroom trip), your expectations as well as preparation of the guide if you are going to be accompanied by one on your trip.

Before you venture on to a psychedelic experience, you (the voyager) need to make some preparations.

- First, understand that the psychedelic experience will be at least a 3-day experience, and not just a one-day trip. The experience will not just begin or end once you consume the magic mushroom and after its effect wears off which is usually 6 to 8 hours maximum. You will continue to observe the effects for a total of 3 days.

- On the first day, try to stay unhurried and quiet. This is the day before you consume the psychedelic mushroom. Do not rush through any task and set aside an hour or two at least for a calm session of deep self-reflection. This is when you should spend time reflecting on your thoughts and analyze them in depth to make sense of them. This helps you better figure out your purpose in life, your life's vision and goals that you genuinely want to set and achieve. You should also spend some part of the day out in a natural setting, a park or a forest or a valley.

- On the second day, you need to use magic mushrooms. Embrace the experience as it happens and sit through with every moment as it occurs. You may feel scared, excited, terrified, happy or just calm - embrace every emotion/feeling as it is and relish it.

- On the third day of the experience, you need to integrate with the experience and take note of the different realizations and discoveries you made.

- On the first day, record your answers to the following questions and go through the same questions on the third day, and compare the findings of the two.

  ✓ What are your preconceived notions regarding psychedelic experiences?

  ✓ What do you think will happen during the trip?

  ✓ What do you expect to experience, learn, resolve, understand and discover?

  ✓ Do you have any spiritual goals? If yes, what are they?

  ✓ What are your psychological goals if any?

  ✓ What are your relationship and social goals if any?

  ✓ Which direction do you want to steer your life to?

  ✓ What truly matters to you?

✓ What do you want to change or improve on in your life?

- In case this is your first time experience with a psychedelic, it is best to have a guide with you. Share your thoughts and findings with him/ her, so he/ she can help you understand your feeling and thoughts better, and clarify any misconceptions or ambiguities you may have regarding the experience. A guide is someone who has prior psychedelic experience, particularly through magic mushrooms. Having a trip with a guide around ensures your safety as he/ she can help you calm down if you feel too upset or are having a bad trip, and can guide you better on how to have a smooth, enjoyable trip.

Setting

The **setting** refers to the surrounding where the trip takes place. It comprises of the physical environment as well as the space where you have the session.

There are primarily two options for a physical setting when you consume a psychedelic.

- A comfortable, clean and uncluttered room having a bed or couch: It is important you have a psychedelic trip in an uncluttered, organized place because if you use it in a cluttered, messy area, the chaos around you will only disturb you mentally. If there is a couch or a bed around, you can comfortably lie down on it when you feel dizzy or sense the trip is taking over your head. You can also have a stereo system or a means to put on music in the room as music in the background is known to enhance the overall psychedelic trip. You need to create a simple, soothing environment that helps you relax and connect better with yourself.

- An outdoor setting you are familiar with: Choosing a familiar setting is a wise move because you feel comfortable in it and can relax better. When choosing an outdoor setting, it is best to stick to one with natural elements such as a park so you connect better with the nature. An outdoor setting usually creates a more exciting, extroverted experience. Even if you plan to use your magic mushrooms outdoors, ensure to take blankets, a couple of pillows and a music player along. You can spread your blanket on the grass or a bench along with a pillow and relax on it while you venture on a psychedelic trip and let its effects wash over your mind.

Whether you plan to have your psychedelic trip indoors or outdoors, take care of the following:

- Wear comfortable clothing so you relax better

- Ensure the setting you choose has a pleasant, comfortable temperature and environment, be it indoors and outdoors.

- Close your eyes and put on some soothing music (this is optional, but recommended) to enhance the experience and engage better with the trip.

- Ensure to choose a place that is not bustling with activity because that can distract and disturb you.

- Pick a peaceful place as a noisy one will only perturb you and interfere with your psychedelic journey.

Substance

This refers to the psychedelic mushroom you are using and the dosage you are consuming.

- If your goal is to use the psychedelic trip to improve your workplace creativity and productivity, a micro-dose of about 0.1 to 0.2g dried magic mushroom works well.

- If you wish to have a mild, entheogenic experience, take a moderate dose comprising of about 1 to 1.5g of dried psilocybin mushrooms. An entheogenic experience is one where you feel united with your body, soul and mind. It is a spiritual and calming experience that enables you to tap into the real you.

- If you aspire to have a great experience where you feel extremely excited and transcend beyond time and space, you should have a high dose comprising of around 2 to 4g of dried magic mushrooms.

It is best not to consume more than 4g of magic mushrooms during any trip because that can lead to intense side effects and mental instability.

Sitter

A sitter or a guide is someone who will take care of you during the trip. He/ she acts as a supportive, reassuring figure throughout your voyage and ensures you do not have a disorienting experience. Besides taking care of you and guiding you, he/ she adjusts the music, manages the setting and ensures you transition through the journey smoothly.

You can find sitters/ guides online by getting in touch with different online forums related to psychedelic mushrooms. These forums can help you find a reliable sitter in your area. You can even reach out to friends and family members who have had prior psychedelic experiences.

That said, if you cannot find a sitter, do not let this glitch deter you from having a psychedelic trip using magic mushrooms. You can go on a psychedelic trip alone too, but in that case, it is best to start off with a very small dose only and stick to it for a few trips till you get the hang of it, and better learn to manage yourself during the trip.

Session

This refers to the overall time for the voyage along with main aspects of it. There are six phases of a psychedelic trip mainly.

- Ingesting the magic mushroom: This is when you consume the chosen dose of your magic mushroom.

- Initial onset: This is when the wave starts to take over you.

- Opening and letting go: This is the phase after a few hours or even a day of ingesting the magic mushroom when you feel free and open, and allow your thoughts to wander away in any direction.

- Plateau: This is when you start to feel stable during the session and settle into the experience. At this point, you acclimatize to the new state of mind and function well with the normal realms of the society. This phase lasts for 2 to 3 hours.

- Gentle Glide: This is when you feel relaxed and calm, and gently move towards the end of the session. This is a good time to carry on with any personal work that you have been meaning to do effectively. You should also go out in the nature and enjoy it.

- End of the session: This usually happens on the third day of the experience, many hours after you ingested the magic mushroom. This is when you need to go through your thoughts and findings, and reflect on them to make better sense of the psychedelic journey.

Situation

This refers to how you, the voyager, integrate the experience into your life. It starts off when the formal 3 day session ends, and spreads on to the following weeks or months right into your future.

Make a conscious effort to think about what matters to you, what you wish to achieve from the experience and how you plan to take that learning forward. Remember not to go overboard with the findings and realizations you make during a psychedelic trip and make life altering decisions based on them.

Take a few weeks to calm down and then make important decisions based on your psychedelic trip and findings such as career shifts, moving to another country, starting a new relationship etc.

If you take care of these 6 S's (5 S's in case you do not have a sitter), you will have an extraordinary, magic experience with the psychedelic mushrooms. It is best to have a single dose and let its effect wear off slowly within 3 to 4 weeks prior to taking another dose. Go slow in the start and once you become comfortable with it, take it frequently.

Conclusion

I hope this guide helps you have a great psychedelic mushroom experience and enjoy their amazing power. Thank you taking out the time to read this book.

Printed in Poland
by Amazon Fulfillment
Poland Sp. z o.o., Wrocław

64235817R00052